Healthy Liver For Life And Cookbook: Breakfast Recipes And More

Learn To Manage Your Nutrition With No Stress - Prevent Cirrhosis And Keep A Healthy Liver

Loren Allen

Healthy Liver For Life And Cookbook

© Copyright 2021 by Loren Allen - All rights reserved.

The following Book is reproduced below with the goal of providing information that is as accurate and reliable as possible. Regardless, purchasing this Book can be seen as consent to the fact that both the publisher and the author of this book are in no way experts on the topics discussed within and that any recommendations or suggestions that are made herein are for entertainment purposes only. Professionals should be consulted as needed prior to undertaking any of the action endorsed herein.

This declaration is deemed fair and valid by both the American Bar Association and the Committee of Publishers Association and is legally binding throughout the United States.

Furthermore, the transmission, duplication, or reproduction of any of the following work including specific information will be considered an illegal act irrespective of if it is done electronically or in print. This extends to creating a secondary or tertiary copy of the work or a recorded copy and is only allowed with the express written consent from the Publisher. All additional right reserved.

Healthy Liver For Life And Cookbook

The information in the following pages is broadly considered a truthful and accurate account of facts and as such, any inattention, use, or misuse of the information in question by the reader will render any resulting actions solely under their purview. There are no scenarios in which the publisher or the original author of this work can be in any fashion deemed liable for any hardship or damages that may befall them after undertaking information described herein.

Additionally, the information in the following pages is intended only for informational purposes and should thus be thought of as universal. As befitting its nature, it is presented without assurance regarding its prolonged validity or interim quality. Trademarks that are mentioned are done without written consent and can in no way be considered an endorsement from the trademark holder.

Table Of Contents

One Of The Most Vital Organs With More Than 500 Functions Known To Date — 8

Tips For People With Liver Cirrhosis Disease — 10

Functions Of The Liver - The Liver: Your Body's Most Important Muscle — 17

Discovering the Stages of Liver Failure — 23

- Liver failure vs. liver disease — 25
- Stages of liver failure — 26
- Causes of liver failure — 28
- Symptoms of acute liver failure — 31
- Symptoms of chronic liver failure — 31
- Diagnosing liver failure — 33
- What are the treatment options for liver failure? — 35
- Preventing liver failure — 37
- Outlook — 38

Healthy Liver For Life And Cookbook

Breakfast Recipes	39
Chilled Green Goddess Soup	39
Beets Omelette	41
Omelette	43
Muffins	44
Cheesy Scrambled Eggs With Fresh Herbs	46
Avocado Crab Omelet	48
Avocado Spread	50
Carrot Omelette	51
Superfood Liver Cleansing Soup	52
Mushroom-egg Casserole	54
Brown Rice Salad	56
Green Salad With Herbs	57
Lemon Muffins	58
Detox Soup	60
Grilled Chicken Salad	62
Peaches Muffins	64
Chili Avocado Scramble	66

Feta And Eggs Mix	68
Overnight Superfood Parfait	69
Quinoa And Potato Bowl	70
Kumquat Muffins	72
Chicken Souvlaki	73
Spiced French Toast	75
Peanut Butter And Cacao Breakfast Quinoa	77
Raspberry Overnight Porridge	79
Herbed Eggs And Mushroom Mix	81
Ham Spinach Ballet	83
Ultimate Liver Detox Soup	84
Breakfast Beans (ful Mudammas)	86
Chicken Stir Fry With Red Onions & Cabbage	88
Chocolate Muffins	90
Deviled Eggs	92
Brown Rice And Grilled Chicken Salad	93
Banana Quinoa	95

Toasted Crostini	97
Quick Cream Of Wheat	99
Pan-fried Chicken With Oregano-orange Chimichurri & Arugula Salad	101
Pineapple, Macha & Beet Chia Pudding	103
Farro Salad	105
Apple Oatmeal	106
Citrus Chicken With Delicious Cold Soup	107
Vegetable Omelet	109
Crunchy Peach, Cranberry And Flax Meal Super Bowl	111
Olive Frittata	113
Pancakes	115
Heavenly Egg Bake With Blackberry	116
Walnuts Yogurt Mix	118
Asparagus With Egg	119
Pear Oatmeal	120
Conclusion	**122**

Healthy Liver For Life And Cookbook

One Of The Most Vital Organs With More Than 500 Functions Known To Date

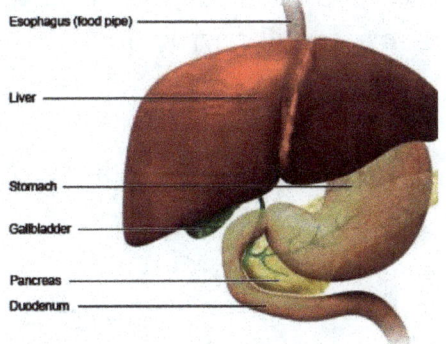

The liver is one of the most vital organs, with more than 500 functions known to date. If your organ's damage from cirrhosis means it can't efficiently perform its duty in getting nutrients out of food and into our bodies for use, a diet tailored specifically towards this ailment may help provide adequate nutrition without over-working what little function you have left. Research has shown that people who are suffering from hepatic diseases like hepatitis or cirrhosis are at risk for complications such as death if they don't receive enough nourishment (emphasis on protein) through their diets; so be sure not to skip meals!

Authors of a 2018 article in the Journal of Clinical Gastroenterology say that "dietary management of cirrhosis is not a one-size-fits-all approach but should be implemented earlier on in the treatment algorithm to improve the clinical prognosis of cirrhosis."

If you have liver cirrhosis, then it's important to stay on top of your diet. If not managed well enough, scarring will continue and worsen which can lead to a number of issues such as an increased risk for cancer or bleeding due to the organ being unable provide blood clotting capability.

If you're concerned about whether managing your diet is something that would be too much trouble for someone with hepatic impairment; don't worry - there are plenty of recipes out there available at any grocery store in most major cities! There should also be information readily available online if one need help finding their way through cooking healthy dishes easily without sacrificing taste.

Tips For People With Liver Cirrhosis Disease

Drinking alcohol and taking medications can cause liver disease to worsen. A healthy diet, like the Mediterranean Diet in combination with a few supplements will help you maintain your weight while limiting complications on the progression of liver disease. You want to avoid high-sugar beverages as well because they are very hard for your body's immune system when it is fighting an infection or just recovering from one!

In short, remember, eat food that is soft, avoid drinking alcohol, don't eat foods that are spicy.

1. Nutrition in Early Liver Cirrhosis Disease

Food

Healthy Liver For Life And Cookbook

A healthy diet should consist of a variety of foods high in nutrients and vitamins. Healthy choices include fruit, vegetables, whole grains, lean protein sources such as chicken breast or tofu, unsalted nuts and seeds like walnuts or almonds for some crunchy texture to your meal on the side. Dairy products provide calcium needed for strong bones but be sure not to add too much fat with milk cheeses because they are higher in saturated fats than low-fat dairy options without cheese that will help keep you full longer after eating them - perfect before bedtime snacks! Keep sodium content lower by avoiding ketchup which is surprisingly one food containing large amounts of salt per serving size at 560mg/1 tbsp., pickles also contain an average 77% more

Selecting foods with healthy fats is important. Choosing unsaturated fats instead of saturated fats and trans fats is a good first step. Unsaturated fats:

- include monosaturated, polyunsaturated and Omega3 fatty acids

- come from plant sources and fish and include avocado, nuts, olive oil, canola oil and safflower oil

- foods high in Omega3 fatty acids include salmon, tuna and mackerel

Beverages

Drink water. Drinking too much sugar is bad for your body and may lead to weight gain or diabetes. Keep in mind that coffee can be good for you, but only up to three cups each day - any more than this could cause a variety of health problems including liver disease like cirrhosis! As always, it's important not to drink alcohol when the goal is improved liver health.

Vitamins and Minerals

Vitamins are the best way to keep you healthy, even if that's all you're eating is a variety of unhealthy foods. One exception would be in cases where someone has alcoholic liver disease and thiamine (vitamin B1), folic acid, and multivitamins should be taken- this includes vitamins B2 and B6 as well. If your diagnosis doesn't include hemochromatosis then vitamin C can also help prevent illness which may arise from an imbalance between iron absorption or retention levels due to genetics or autoimmune conditions such as celiac disease .

Vitamins provide much needed nutrients for many people who might not otherwise get them through their diet alone! An example would be those with alcohol related liver diseases; they

2. Nutrition in Advanced Liver Cirrhosis Disease

Food

      Poor appetite, nausea and vomiting can lead to malnutrition in advanced liver disease (ALD). Loss of protein from decreased absorption or increased losses also contribute. Protein is not restricted even with ALD but you should avoid large amounts due the fact that your body does not store it well. Eating small meals more frequently may be better tolerated by an individual with ALD since they are much easier for their now-defunct liver to process than larger ones would be at one sitting time per day--this will also help keep them feeling full longer!

ALD causes the kidneys to hold sodium (salt) which then results in your body holding more fluid thus increasing ascites (swollen abdomen) and swelling of the hands, legs and feet. Your provider may ask that you restrict your sodium intake to 2000 mg or less (1 teaspoon of salt contains approximately 2300mg sodium). Sodium in all foods and beverages must be calculated into this amount. Reading sodium content on packaging will be necessary. You should remember that the sodium content on the package is for the serving size indicated on the label, not for the entire amount of the package. If you have chronic kidney disease, salt substitutes should be avoided because they are high in potassium.

Beverages

Your provider will tell you if or when to restrict your fluid intake with liver disease. The goal is 1500-2000 ml per day, but more than that can be prescribed by a doctor in order alleviate symptoms of feeling thirsty which could stem from taking diuretics (water pills). One way to keep track of how much water you drink for the whole day would be filling up one pitcher and every time we drink something take out an equivalent amount of water so it never goes below this limit! If on a restricted diet due to being on these medications, there are tricks such as drinking soup instead because they still count towards the daily total. Sugar-free frozen pops, sugar-free sour candy, sugar-free gelatin, sucking on lemon or lime slices and eating ice cold fruit and vegetables will help relieve thirst. Frozen grapes are a good option. Fluid from the sugar-free frozen pops and gelatin must be included in the daily allowance of fluid intake, as will the fluid in juicy fruit like watermelon.

Vitamins and Minerals

There is a fine line between not enough and too much when taking vitamin supplements. When you are sick, it may be difficult to know what the right amount of vitamins for your illness might be if you aren't sure of their effects on an already broken system. For example, excessive amounts can injure your liver which is at risk in this case because they have also been depleted from other illnesses such as Jaundice (yellow skin and eyes).

Fatigue, muscle weakness and twitches and cramps of your arms, hands and feet may indicate magnesium deficiency in ALD. Your provider may order a blood test to determine magnesium level and, if low, a supplement will be ordered. ALD may also cause a zinc deficiency. Signs of a zinc deficiency include decreased appetite, decreased ability to fight infection, diarrhea and hair loss. A zinc supplement may be ordered by your provider. Muscle cramps can also be relieved with drinking either regular or diet tonic water because of the quinine content. It is important not to drink more than 4 ounces per day because of the high sodium content.

Functions Of The Liver - The Liver: Your Body's Most Important Muscle

The liver is the largest organ in your body and without it life would be impossible. The liver's job includes filtering blood, maintaining healthy sugar levels, regulating clotting of blood (which prevents you from bleeding excessively), and performing hundreds more tasks that keep us alive. Located just under our ribs on the right side of our abdomen, this most important muscle helps fight infection by making new cells to replace dying ones!

Key Facts

The liver filters all of the blood in the body and breaks down poisonous substances, such as alcohol and drugs.

The liver also produces bile, a fluid that helps digest fats and carry away waste.

The liver consists of four lobes, which are each made up of eight sections and thousands of lobules (or small lobes).

Functions of the Liver

The liver is the body's trash compactor, producing essential blood sugars and nutrients. It also removes waste products from your bloodstream to provide you with a squeaky-clean circulatory system!

A lot of people might not be aware that their liver does so much work for them every day, but it really can't do everything without some help or support either - just like any other muscle in your body needs extra care when tired after working out. That said, there are healthy diet options to give yourself an energy boost so that this important organ doesn't have as tough a time performing its functions throughout the course of our 24 hour lifespan.

Albumin Production: Albumin is a protein that keeps fluids in the bloodstream from leaking into surrounding tissue. It also carries hormones, vitamins, and enzymes through the body.

Bile Production: Bile is a fluid that is critical to the digestion and absorption of fats in the small intestine.

Filters Blood: All the blood leaving the stomach and intestines passes through the liver, which removes toxins, byproducts, and other harmful substances.

Regulates Amino Acids: The production of proteins depend on amino acids. The liver makes sure amino acid levels in the bloodstream remain healthy.

Regulates Blood Clotting: Blood clotting coagulants are created using vitamin K, which can only be absorbed with the help of bile, a fluid the liver produces.

Resists Infections: As part of the filtering process, the liver also removes bacteria from the bloodstream.

Stores Vitamins and Minerals: The liver stores significant amounts of vitamins A, D, E, K, and B12, as well as iron and copper.

Processes Glucose: The liver removes excess glucose (sugar) from the bloodstream and stores it as glycogen. As needed, it can convert glycogen back into glucose.

Anatomy of the Liver

The liver is reddish-brown and shaped approximately like a cone or a wedge, with the small end above the spleen and stomach and the large end above the small intestine. The entire organ is located below the lungs in the right upper abdomen. It weighs between 3 and 3.5 pounds.

Structure

The liver is a large organ that consists of four lobes. The two larger, right lobe and left lobe are divided by the falciform ligament, which connects the liver to the abdominal wall. These segments can be further subdivided into eight smaller ones each with its own ducts for bile (a digestive fluid).

Parts

The following are some of the most important individual parts of the liver:

Common Hepatic Duct: A tube that carries bile out of the liver. It is formed from the intersection of the right and left hepatic ducts.

Falciform Ligament: A thin, fibrous ligament that separates the two lobes of the liver and connects it to the abdominal wall.

Glisson's Capsule: A layer of loose connective tissue that surrounds the liver and its related arteries and ducts.

Hepatic Artery: The main blood vessel that supplies the liver with oxygenated blood.

Hepatic Portal Vein: The blood vessel that carries blood from the gastrointestinal tract, gallbladder, pancreas, and spleen to the liver.

Lobes: The anatomical sections of the liver.

Lobules: Microscopic building blocks of the liver.

Peritoneum: A membrane covering the liver that forms the exterior.

Maintaining a Healthy Liver

Healthy Liver For Life And Cookbook

The best way to avoid liver disease is by taking active steps towards a healthy life. The following are some recommendations that will help keep the liver functioning as it should:

Avoid Illicit Drugs: Illicit drugs are toxins that the liver must filter out. Taking these drugs can cause long-term damage.

Drink Alcohol Moderately: Alcohol must be broken down by the liver. While the liver can moderate amounts, excessive alcohol use can cause damage.

Exercise Regularly: A regular exercise routine will help promote general health for every organ, including the liver.

Eat Healthy Foods: Eating excessive fats can make it difficult for the liver to function and lead to fatty liver disease.

Practice Safe Sex: Use protection to avoid sexually transmitted diseases such as hepatitis C.

Vaccinate: Especially when traveling, get appropriate vaccinations against hepatitis A and B, as well as diseases such as malaria and yellow fever, which grow in the liver.

Discovering the Stages of Liver Failure

Liver failure is a life-threatening emergency. The two main types of liver failures are acute or chronic and it can either come on quickly, like when one has an infection that leads to increased alcohol abuse or if you're born with certain genetics (such as hemochromatosis), whereas the other type occurs gradually over time in some people who may not have any risks factors for developing their disease but just develop them due to lifestyle choices.

Acute liver failure suddenly comes on while chronic cases happen slowly over weeks/months so they're easier treated before serious damage happens; however, this doesn't mean your symptoms will go away because there's no cure--only treatments--and many sufferers don't know about early signs which could be monitored.

The liver is an important part of the body. It can be damaged and not work properly. The damage can happen in stages that get worse over time.

Stages of liver failure

Inflammation. In this early stage, the liver is enlarged or inflamed.

Fibrosis. Scar tissue begins to replace healthy tissue in the inflamed liver.

Cirrhosis. Severe scarring has built up, making it difficult for the liver to function properly.

End-stage liver disease (ESLD). Liver function has deteriorated to the point where the damage can't be reversed other than with a liver transplant.

Liver cancer. The development and multiplication of unhealthy cells in the liver can occur at any stage of liver failure, although people with cirrhosis are more at risk.

Liver failure vs. liver disease

The liver is one of the most important organs in your body. There are many different types of diseases that can affect it, but two specific ones to watch out for are degenerative and acute hepatitis. The first usually causes damage over time while the latter often occurs quickly due to rapid infection or injury from an outside source like alcohol abuse or a car accident. These conditions result in inflammation, pain, swelling and even death if left untreated! It's good you know what these look like so when they come up on your medical tests you'll be able to react appropriately instead of waiting around until something more serious happens again later down the line.

Stages of liver failure

Damage from liver disease can happen in stages. The damage goes up and it makes the liver not work as well.

Inflammation

In this early stage, your liver becomes swollen or inflamed. Many people with this condition do not have symptoms. If it continues for a long time, your liver can be permanently damaged.

Fibrosis

Fibrosis is inflammation of the liver. This can happen when the liver starts to scar.

The scar tissue that's generated in this stage replaces healthy liver tissue. But the scarred tissue can't do what the healthy tissue did. It can start to affect your liver's ability to work right.

Fibrosis is hard to notice because there are not usually any symptoms.

Cirrhosis

When you have cirrhosis, your liver is damaged. That means it doesn't work as well.

When you first get liver disease, you may not have any symptoms. But now, you might start to feel bad.

End-stage liver disease (ESLD)

People with ESLD have a disease called cirrhosis. This means that the liver has been damaged.

ESLD is associated with complications such as ascites and hepatic encephalopathy. It can't be reversed unless you get a liver transplant.

Liver cancer

Cancer is when cells in your body are not healthy. If you have cancer in your liver, it is called primary liver cancer.

Although it can happen at any stage of liver failure, people with cirrhosis are more likely to get liver cancer.

Some common symptoms of liver cancer include:

- unexplained weight loss
- abdominal pain or swelling
- loss of appetite or feeling full after eating a small amount of food
- nausea or vomiting
- yellowing of the skin and eyes (jaundice)
- skin itching

Causes of liver failure

The cause of liver failure can depend on the type of liver failure — acute or chronic.

Causes of acute liver failure

Acute liver failure occurs quickly. It can be caused by many things, but sometimes the exact cause is unknown.. Some possible causes include:

- A viral infection happens when a virus enters the body. There are three viruses that can cause infections: hepatitis A, B, or E.
- A person might overdose on acetaminophen (Tylenol) if they take too much.
- There are many different reactions to prescription medicines. For example, some people might have a reaction when they use antibiotics, NSAIDs or anti-epileptic drugs.
- Reactions to herbal supplements, such as ma huang and kava kava.
- metabolic conditions, such as Wilson's disease
- autoimmune conditions are when your body attacks itself. For example, there is autoimmune hepatitis.
- If you have the condition where the veins of your liver are affected, like Budd-Chiari syndrome, then it is important to eat less fat.
- Exposure to toxins can happen in the workplace or when you eat a bad mushroom.

Causes of chronic liver failure

Liver failure happens when a person's liver gets hurt over time. This can lead to cirrhosis, which is when there is too much scar tissue on the liver and it stops working right.

Some examples of possible causes of cirrhosis include:

- chronic hepatitis B or C infection
- Alcohol-related liver disease (ARLD) is a disease that can happen when you drink alcohol. It happens in your liver.
- Nonalcoholic fatty liver disease means that someone has a lot of fat in their liver and they do not drink alcohol.
- autoimmune hepatitis
- Diseases that affect your bile duct can be very bad. They are called cholangitis.

Symptoms of acute liver failure

Acute liver failure can happen to people who do not have a condition in their liver. This is an emergency and people should see a doctor when they have symptoms that are like acute liver failure.

The symptoms of acute liver failure can include:

- feeling unwell (malaise)
- feeling tired or sleepy
- nausea or vomiting
- abdominal pain or swelling
- yellowing of the skin and eyes (jaundice)
- feeling confused or disoriented

Symptoms of chronic liver failure

Some symptoms of chronic liver failure are early symptoms and some are more advanced. Early symptoms may include:

- feeling tired or fatigued
- loss of appetite
- nausea or vomiting
- mild abdominal discomfort or pain

Some symptoms that might mean you have a liver problem are:

- yellowing of the skin and eyes (jaundice)
- easy bruising or bleeding
- feeling confused or disoriented
- buildup of fluid in your abdomen, arms, or legs
- darkening of your urine
- severe skin itching

Diagnosing liver failure

To diagnose liver failure, your doctor will start by taking your medical history and performing a physical examination. They may then perform additional tests to rule out other causes of symptoms such as: blood work-up for anemia or anaemia; chest X-ray to look at the lungs and heart health; EKG for an irregular heartbeat (arrhythmia); urinalysis looking at kidney function along with electrolytes in urine samples.; imaging scans like ultrasounds or CTs which can visualize different parts of our body.

You might also have some generalized pain around the abdomen area that you'll need to mention on this list too!

- A **liver blood test** is a test to see how your liver is working. There are different proteins and enzymes in the blood, and these can tell.
- **Other blood tests.** Your doctor can do a blood test to see if you have any problems in your liver. There are many different tests that they can do.
- **Imaging tests.** Ultrasound, CT scan, and MRI can help your doctor to see your liver.
- **Biopsy.** Taking a tissue sample of your liver can help your doctor see if there is scar tissue or other reasons for your condition.

What are the treatment options for liver failure?

The liver is important for our body. We need it to help us do things like digest food, and if it doesn't work, then we will have a problem. If there is something going wrong with our liver, then we might have to take medicine or get surgery so that the damage can stop happening.

For example, antiviral medications can be used to treat a viral hepatitis infection, or immune suppressing medication can be given to treat autoimmune hepatitis.

Lifestyle changes may also be recommended as a part of your treatment. These can include things like abstaining from alcohol, losing weight, or avoiding the use of certain medications.

The American Liver Foundation estimates that a large percentage of the damage to your liver can be reversed, if caught and treated. If not, this may lead to cirrhosis or ESLD which is often irreversible but sometimes slows down progression.

What about acute liver failure?

Acute liver failure is often treated in the intensive care unit of a hospital. Supportive care can be given to help stabilize your condition and control any complications during treatment and recovery from acute liver failure.

A medication overdose or reaction may also lead you to receive drugs that reverse its effects, while a potential indication for transplantation may exist for some people with this type of serious medical emergency due to their severe illness severity, which could even progress into coma if left untreated too long!

Preventing liver failure

You can help to prevent liver failure by making lifestyle changes. If you make them, your liver will be happy and healthy. Here are some tips for improving liver health:

- Drink alcohol in moderation, and never mix medications with alcohol.
- Take medications only when needed, and carefully follow any dosing instructions.
- Don't mix medications without first consulting your doctor.
- To maintain a healthy weight, there is a connection to liver disease.
- Get vaccinated against hepatitis A and B.
- Be sure to have regular physicals with your doctor during which they perform liver blood tests.

Outlook

Liver failure is when your liver can't function properly. It can be either acute or chronic, and in the later stages of life it may require a transplant to save lives. Liver deterioration could have been caused by alcoholism, hepatitis-C infection, cancer treatment side effects such as chemotherapy drugs that damage the healthy cells along with tumor cells; or even radiation for kidney stones where some parts of belly will get more exposed than others due to increased urination which was previously being handled by kidneys before they were damaged from stone disease - you name it! In any case though whether its just one factor like alcohol abuse leading up to cirrhosis and then eventually hepatocellular carcinoma (liver cancer) if untreated through surgery followed.

People who are diagnosed with liver disease are often monitored throughout their life to make sure that their condition isn't worsening or causing further liver damage. If you have concerns about liver health or about liver failure, be sure to talk to your doctor.

Breakfast Recipes

Chilled Green Goddess Soup

Servings: 3

Cooking Time: 10 Minutes

Ingredients:

- 6 cups cucumber
- 2 stalks celery chopped
- 1-2 cups water (depending how thin you want it)
- 2 tablespoons fresh lime juice
- 1 cup watercress leaves
- 1 cup rocket leaves
- ½ cup mashed avocado (roughly 1 avocado)
- 1 teaspoon wheatgrass power or a mixed green powder, optional
- Sea salt to tast

Directions:

- Blend all ingredients except the avocado in a blender until a broth forms. Strain the liquid through a cheesecloth or fine sieve. Then return to blender and add the avocado and blend until smooth.
- Garnish with a few watercress leaves and cracked black pepper.

Nutrition:

283.6 Calories 11.5g fat 31g carbs 10.9g protein

Beets Omelette

Servings:1

Cooking Time:10 Minutes

Ingredients:

- 2 eggs
- ¼ tsp salt
- ¼ tsp black pepper
- 1 tablespoon olive oil
- ¼ cup cheese
- ¼ tsp basil
- 1 cup beets

Directions:

- In a bowl combine all ingredients together and mix well
- In a skillet heat olive oil and pour the egg mixture
- Cook for 1-2 minutes per side
- When ready remove omelette from the skillet and serve

Nutrition:

50g carbs 11g fat 10g protein 320 Calories

Omelette

Servings: 4

Cooking Time: 15 Minutes

Ingredients:

- 2 eggs
- ¼ tsp salt
- ¼ tsp black pepper
- 1 tablespoon olive oil
- ¼ cup cheese
- ¼ tsp basil

Directions:

- In a bowl combine all ingredients together and mix well
- In a skillet heat olive oil and pour the egg mixture
- Cook for 1-2 minutes per side
- When ready remove omelette from the skillet and serve

Nutrition:

2g carbs 6g fat 10g protein 100 Calories

Muffins

Servings:4

Cooking Time:20 Minutes

Ingredients:

- 2 eggs
- 1 tablespoon olive oil
- 1 cup milk
- 2 cups whole wheat flour
- 1 tsp baking soda
- ¼ tsp baking soda
- 1 tsp cinnamon

Directions:

- In a bowl combine all wet ingredients
- In another bowl combine all dry ingredients
- Combine wet and dry ingredients together
- Pour mixture into 8-12 preparation ared muffin cups, fill 2/3 of the cups
- Bake for 18-20 minutes at 375 F
- When ready remove from the oven and serve

Nutrition:

2g carbs 6g fat 10g protein 100 Calories

Cheesy Scrambled Eggs With Fresh Herbs

Servings: 4

Cooking Time: 10 Minutes

Ingredients:

- Eggs – 3
- Egg whites – 2
- Cream cheese – ½ cup
- Unsweetened rice milk – ¼ cup
- Chopped scallion – 1 Tablespoon green part only
- Chopped fresh tarragon – 1 Tablespoon
- Unsalted butter – 2 Tablespoons.
- Ground black pepper to taste

Directions:

- In a container, mix the eggs, egg whites, cream cheese, rice milk, scallions, and tarragon until mixed and smooth.
- Melt the butter in a skillet.
- Pour in the egg mix and cook, stirring, for 5 minutes or until the eggs are thick and curds creamy.
- Season with pepper and serve.

Nutrition:

Calories: 221 ,Fat: 19g ,Carb: 3g ,Phosphorus: 119mg ,Potassium: 140mg ,Sodium: 193mg ,Protein: 8g

Avocado Crab Omelet

Servings:2

Cooking Time:10 Minutes

Ingredients:

- 1/4 pound crab meat
- 4 large free-range eggs, beaten
- 1/2 medium avocado, diced
- 1 medium tomato, diced
- 1 teaspoon olive oil
- 1/8 teaspoon freshly ground black pepper
- A pinch of salt
- 1 tablespoon freshly chopped cilantro

Directions:

- Cook crab in a skillet following the instructions on the packet; chop the cooked crab and set aside.
- In a small bowl, toss together avocado, tomato, and cilantro; season with sea salt and pepper and set aside.

- In a separate bowl, beat the eggs and set aside.
- Set a skillet over medium heat; add olive oil and heat until hot.
- Add half of the egg to the skillet and tilt the skillet to cover the bottom. When almost cooked, add crab onto one side of the egg and fold in half. Cook for 1 minute more and top with the avocado-tomato mixture.
- Repeat with the remaining ingredients for the second omelet.

Nutrition:

242 Calories 7g Carbs 19g Fat 12g Protein

Avocado Spread

Servings: 8

Cooking Time: 10 Minutes

Ingredients:

- 2 avocados, peeled, pitted and roughly chopped
- 1 tablespoon sun-dried tomatoes, chopped
- 2 tablespoons lemon juice
- 3 tablespoons cherry tomatoes, chopped
- ¼ cup red onion, chopped
- 1 teaspoon oregano, dried
- 2 tablespoons parsley, chopped
- 4 kalamata olives, pitted and chopped
- A pinch of salt and black pepper

Directions:

- Put the avocados in a bowl and mash with a fork.
- Add the rest of the ingredients, stir to combine and serve as a morning spread.

Nutrition:

calories 110, fat 10, fiber 3.8, carbs 5.7, protein 1.2

Carrot Omelette

Servings: 4

Cooking Time: 20 Minutes

Ingredients:

- 2 eggs
- ¼ tsp salt
- ¼ tsp black pepper
- 1 tablespoon olive oil
- ¼ cup cheese
- ¼ tsp basil
- 1 cup carrot

Directions:

- In a bowl combine all ingredients together and mix well
- In a skillet heat olive oil and pour the egg mixture
- Cook for 1-2 minutes per side
- When ready remove omelette from the skillet and serv

Nutrition:

50g carbs 11g fat 10g protein 320 Calories

Superfood Liver Cleansing Soup

Servings:3

Cooking Time:20 Minutes

Ingredients:

- 1/4 cup water
- 2 cloves garlic, minced
- 1/2 of a red onion, diced
- 1 tablespoon fresh ginger, peeled and minced
- 1 cup chopped tomatoes
- 1 small head of broccoli, florets
- 3 medium carrots, diced
- 3 celery stalks, diced
- 6 cups water
- 1/4 teaspoon cinnamon
- 1 teaspoon turmeric
- 1/8 teaspoon cayenne pepper
- Freshly ground black pepper
- juice of 1 lemon
- 1 cup purple cabbage, chopped
- 2 cups kale, torn in pieces

Directions:

- Bring a large pot of water to a gentle boil over medium heat. Add garlic and onion and cook for about 2 minutes, stirring occasionally.
- Stir in carrots, broccoli, tomatoes, fresh ginger, celery and cook for another 3 minutes. Stir in cayenne, turmeric, cinnamon, and black pepper.
- Add half cup of water to the pot and bring to a gentle boil; lower heat and simmer until the veggies and tender, for about 15 minutes.
- Stir in kale, cabbage, and fresh lemon juice during the last 2 minutes of cooking. Serve hot or warm.

Nutrition:

283.6 Calories 11.5g fat 31g carbs 10.9g protein

Mushroom-egg Casserole

Servings:3

Cooking Time:30 Minutes

Ingredients:

- ½ cup mushrooms, chopped
- ½ yellow onion, diced
- 4 eggs, beaten
- 1 tablespoon coconut flakes
- ½ teaspoon chili pepper
- 1 oz Cheddar cheese, shredded
- 1 teaspoon canola oil

Directions:

- Pour canola oil in the skillet and preheat well.
- Add mushrooms and onion and roast for 5-8 minutes or until the vegetables are light brown.
- Transfer the cooked vegetables in the casserole mold.
- Add coconut flakes, chili pepper, and Cheddar cheese.
- Then add eggs and stir well.
- Bake the casserole for 15 minutes at 360F

Nutrition:

Calories 152, fat 11.1, fiber 0.7, carbs 3, protein 10.4

Brown Rice Salad

Servings: 4

Cooking Time: 10 Minutes

Ingredients:

- 9 ounces brown rice, cooked
- 7 cups baby arugula
- 15 ounces canned garbanzo beans, drained and rinsed
- 4 ounces feta cheese, crumbled
- ¾ cup basil, chopped
- A pinch of salt and black pepper
- 2 tablespoons lemon juice
- ¼ teaspoon lemon zest, grated
- ¼ cup olive oil

Directions:

In a salad bowl, combine the brown rice with the arugula, the beans and the rest of the ingredients, toss and serve cold for breakfast.

Nutrition:

calories 473, fat 22, fiber 7, carbs 53, protein 13

Green Salad With Herbs

Servings:4

Cooking Time:30 Minutes

Ingredients:

- 1 bunch rocket
- 2 baby cos, outer leaves discarded, roughly chopped
- 1 curly endive, outer leaves removed, roughly chopped
- 2 tablespoons chopped parsley
- 2 tablespoons chopped fresh dill
- 2 tablespoons snipped chives
- 1/2 cup extra-virgin olive oil
- 2 tablespoons fresh lemon juice

Directions:

- In a large bowl, mix rocket, cos and endive and herbs.
- In another small bowl, whisk together olive oil, fresh lemon juice, salt and pepper until well blended; pour over the salad and toss to coat well. Serve.

Nutrition:

283.6 Calories 11.5g fat 31g carbs 10.9g protein

Lemon Muffins

Servings: 4

Cooking Time: 30 Minutes

Ingredients:

- 2 eggs
- 1 tablespoon olive oil
- 1 cup milk
- 2 cups whole wheat flour
- 1 tsp baking soda
- ¼ tsp baking soda
- 1 tsp cinnamon
- 1 cup lemon slices

Directions:

- In a bowl combine all wet ingredients
- In another bowl combine all dry ingredients
- Combine wet and dry ingredients together
- Pour mixture into 8-12 preparation ared muffin cups, fill 2/3 of the cups
- Bake for 18-20 minutes at 375 F
- When ready remove from the oven and serve

Nutrition:

2g carbs 6g fat 10g protein 100 Calories

Detox Soup

Servings:3

Cooking Time:40 Minutes

Ingredients:

- 4 cloves garlic, crushed
- 2 medium leeks, chopped
- 1 serrano pepper, thinly sliced
- 4 celery stalks, chopped
- 4 carrots, diced
- 3 rutabagas, peeled and diced
- 8 cups water
- 2 cups pinto beans, cooked with cooking liquids
- 3 tomatoes, diced
- 3 zucchini, diced
- 2 bunches kale, thinly sliced
- 3 tablespoons lemon juice
- Sea salt
- Freshly cracked black pepper

Directions:

- Heat a pot over medium heat; add garlic, leeks, and serranoes. Cook for about 5 minutes, stirring.
- Add celery, carrots, and rutabagas; cook for about 3 minutes more and stir in water, pinto beans, and tomatoes; simmer for about 30 minutes or until the beans are cooked through.
- Stir in zucchini and kale, 15 minutes before serving. Remove from heat and stir in lemon juice; season with sea salt and black pepper and serve.

Nutrition:

283.6 Calories 11.5g fat 31g carbs 10.9g protein

Grilled Chicken Salad

Servings: 2

Cooking Time: 20 Minutes

Ingredients:

- 4 cups chopped broccoli
- 1/4 cup extra virgin olive oil
- 1/2 small red onion, thinly sliced
- 1 carrot, coarsely grated
- 4 chicken thighs, skinless
- 1 1/2 tablespoons Cajun seasoning
- 1/4 cup lemon juice
- 1 tablespoon drained baby capers
- 1 lemon, cut into wedges, to serve

Directions:

- Drizzle chicken with oil and sprinkle with seasoning; rub to coat well.
- Heat your grill to medium heat and grill the chicken for about 8 minutes per side or until cooked through and golden browned on the outside.
- In the meantime, place the grated broccoli in a bowl and add in red onion, carrots, capers, lime juice and the remaining oil, salt and pepper; toss to combine well and serve with grilled chicken garnished with lemon wedges.

Nutrition:

283.6 Calories 11.5g fat 31g carbs 10.9g protein

Peaches Muffins

Servings:4

Cooking Time:30 Minutes

Ingredients:

- 2 eggs
- 1 tablespoon olive oil
- 1 cup milk
- 2 cups whole wheat flour
- 1 tsp baking soda
- ¼ tsp baking soda
- 1 cup peaches
- 1 tsp cinnamon
- ¼ cup molasses

Directions:

- In a bowl combine all wet ingredients
- In another bowl combine all dry ingredients
- Combine wet and dry ingredients together
- Pour mixture into 8-12 preparation ared muffin cups, fill 2/3 of the cups
- Bake for 18-20 minutes at 375 F, when ready remove and serve

Nutrition:

2g carbs 6g fat 10g protein 100 Calories

Chili Avocado Scramble

Servings:4

Cooking Time:0 Minutes

Ingredients:

- 4 eggs, beaten
- 1 white onion, diced
- 1 tablespoon avocado oil
- 1 avocado, finely chopped
- ½ teaspoon chili flakes
- 1 oz Cheddar cheese, shredded
- ½ teaspoon salt
- 1 tablespoon fresh parsley

Directions:

- Pour avocado oil in the skillet and bring it to boil.
- Then add diced onion and roast it until it is light brown.
- Meanwhile, mix up together chili flakes, beaten eggs, and salt.
- Pour the egg mixture over the cooked onion and cook the mixture for 1 minute over the medium heat.
- After this, scramble the eggs well with the help of the fork or spatula. Cook the eggs until they are solid but soft.
- After this, add chopped avocado and shredded cheese.
- Stir the scramble well and transfer in the serving plates.
- Sprinkle the meal with fresh parsley

Nutrition:

calories 236, fat 20.1, fiber 4, carbs 7.4, protein 8.6

Feta And Eggs Mix

Servings: 4

Cooking Time: 5 Minutes

Directions:

- Melt butter in the skillet and add beaten eggs.
- Then add parsley, salt, and scrambled eggs. Cook the eggs for 1 minute over the high heat.
- Add ground black pepper and scramble eggs with the help of the fork.
- Cook the eggs for 3 minutes over the medium-high heat

Nutrition:

calories 110, fat 8.4, fiber 0.1, carbs 1.1, protein 7.6

Overnight Superfood Parfait

Servings: 3

Cooking Time: 10 Minutes

Ingredients:

- 1 cup almond milk
- 1 teaspoon spirulina powder
- 1 teaspoon raw honey
- 4 tablespoons chia seeds
- 4 tablespoons Greek yogurt, to serve
- 1 cup fresh cranberries, to serve
- 1 cup fresh blueberries
- 1 cup toasted almonds

Directions:

1. In a bowl, mix together all the ingredients until well combined; let set for overnight. To serve, add half of the yogurt in a serving glass and top with a third of berries and toasted almonds; repeat the layers until the glass is full. Enjoy!

Nutrition:

242 Calories 7g Carbs 19g Fat 12g Protein

Quinoa And Potato Bowl

Servings: 4

Cooking Time: 20 Minutes

Ingredients:

- 1 sweet potato, peeled, chopped
- 1 tablespoon olive oil
- ½ teaspoon chili flakes
- ½ teaspoon salt
- 1 cup quinoa
- 2 cups of water
- 1 teaspoon butter
- 1 tablespoon fresh cilantro, chopped

Directions:

- Line the baking tray with parchment.
- Arrange the chopped sweet potato in the tray and sprinkle it with chili flakes, salt, and olive oil.
- Bake the sweet potato for 20 minutes at 355F.
- Meanwhile, pour water in the saucepan.
- Add quinoa and cook it over the medium heat for 7 minutes or until quinoa will absorb all liquid.
- Add butter in the cooked quinoa and stir well.
- Transfer it in the bowls, add baked sweet potato and chopped cilantro

Nutrition:

calories 221, fat 7.1, fiber 3.9, carbs 33.2, protein 6.6

Kumquat Muffins

Servings:4

Cooking Time:30 Minutes

Ingredients:

- 2 eggs
- 1 tablespoon olive oil
- 1 cup milk
- 2 cups whole wheat flour
- 1 tsp baking soda
- ¼ tsp baking soda
- 1 tsp cinnamon
- 1 cup kumquat
- In a bowl combine all wet ingredients
- In another bowl combine all dry ingredients
- Combine wet and dry ingredients together
- Pour mixture into 8-12 preparation ared muffin cups, fill 2/3 of the cups
- Bake for 18-20 minutes at 375 F
- When ready remove from the oven and serve

Nutrition:

2g carbs 6g fat 10g protein 100 Calorie

Chicken Souvlaki

Servings:4

Cooking Time:2 Minutes

Ingredients:

- 4 pieces (6-inch) pitas, cut into halves
- 2 cups roasted chicken breast skinless, boneless, and sliced
- 1/4 cup red onion, thinly sliced
- 1/2 teaspoon dried oregano
- 1/2 cup Greek yogurt, plain
- 1/2 cup plum tomato, chopped
- 1/2 cup cucumber, peeled, chopped
- 1/2 cup (2 ounces) feta cheese, crumbled
- 1 tablespoon olive oil, extra-virgin, divided
- 1 tablespoon fresh dill, chopped
- 1 cup iceberg lettuce, shredded
- 1 1/4 teaspoons minced garlic, bottled, divided

Directions:

- In a small mixing bowl, combine the yogurt, cheese, 1 teaspoon of the olive oil, and 1/4 teaspoon of the garlic until well mixed.
- In a large skillet, heat the remaining olive oil over medium-high heat. Add the remaining 1 teaspoon garlic and the oregano; sauté for 20 seconds.
- Add the chicken; cook for about 2 minutes or until the chicken are heated through.
- Put 1/4 cup chicken into each pita halves. Top with 2 tablespoons yogurt mix, 2 tablespoons lettuce, 1 tablespoon tomato, and 1 tablespoon cucumber. Divide the onion between the pita halves.

Nutrition:

414 Cal, 13.7 g total fat (6.4 g sat. fat, 1.4 g poly. Fat, 4.7 g mono), 81 mg chol., 595 mg sodium, 38 g carb., 2 g fiber, 32.3 g protein.

Spiced French Toast

Servings: 4

Cooking Time: 12 Minutes

Ingredients:

- 4 eggs
- ½ cup Homemade Rice Milk (here, or use unsweetened store-bought) or almond milk
- ¼ cup freshly squeezed orange juice
- 1 teaspoon ground cinnamon
- ½ teaspoon ground ginger
- Pinch ground cloves
- 1 tablespoon unsalted butter, divided
- 8 slices white bread

Directions:

- Whisk eggs, rice milk, orange juice, cinnamon, ginger, and cloves until well blended in a large bowl.
- Melt half the butter in a large skillet. It should be in medium-high heat only.
- Dredge four of the bread slices in the egg mixture until well soaked, and place them in the skillet.
- Cook the toast until golden brown on both sides, turning once, about 6 minutes total.
- Repeat with the remaining butter and bread.
- Serve 2 pieces of hot French toast to each person.

Nutrition:

Calories: 236; Total fat: 11g; Saturated fat: 4g; Cholesterol: 220mg; Sodium: 84mg; Carbohydrates: 27g; Fiber: 1g; Phosphorus: 119mg; Potassium: 158mg; Protein: 11g

Peanut Butter And Cacao Breakfast Quinoa

Servings:1

Cooking Time:10 Minutes

Ingredients:

- 1/3 cup quinoa flakes
- 1/2 cup unsweetened nondairy milk,
- 1/2 cup of water
- 1/8 cup raw cacao powder
- One tablespoon natural creamy peanut butter
- 1/8 teaspoon ground cinnamon
- One banana, mashed
- Fresh berries of choice, for serving
- Chopped nuts of choice, for servin

Directions:

- Using an 8-quart pot over medium-high heat, stir together the quinoa flakes, milk, water, cacao powder, peanut butter, and cinnamon. Cook and stir it until the mixture begins to simmer. Turn the heat to medium-low and cook for 3 to 5 minutes, stirring frequently.
- Stir in the bananas and cook until hot.
- Serve topped with fresh berries, nuts, and a splash of milk

Nutrition:

Calories: 471 ,Fat: 16g ,Protein: 18g ,Carbohydrates: 69g ,Fiber: 16g

Raspberry Overnight Porridge

Servings: 12

Cooking Time: 20 Minute

Ingredients:

- ⅓ cup of rolled oats
- ½ cup almond milk
- 1 tablespoon of honey
- 5-6 raspberries, fresh or canned and unsweetened
- ⅓ cup of rolled oats
- ½ cup almond milk
- 1 tablespoon of honey
- 5-6 raspberries, fresh or canned and unsweetened

Directions:

- Combine the oats, almond milk, and honey in a mason jar and place into the fridge for overnight.
- Serve the next morning with the raspberries on top.

Nutrition:

Healthy Liver For Life And Cookbook

Calories: 143.6 kcal ,Carbohydrate: 34.62 g ,Protein: 3.44 g ,Sodium: 77.88 mg ,Potassium: 153.25 mg ,Phosphorus: 99.3 mg ,Dietary Fiber: 7.56 g ,Fat: 3.91 g

Herbed Eggs And Mushroom Mix

Servings:4

Cooking Time:20 Minutes

Ingredients:

- 1 red onion, chopped
- 1 bell pepper, chopped
- 1 tablespoon tomato paste
- 1/3 cup water
- ½ teaspoon of sea salt
- 1 tablespoon butter
- 1 cup cremini mushrooms, chopped
- 1 tablespoon fresh parsley
- 1 tablespoon fresh dill
- 1 teaspoon dried thyme
- ½ teaspoon dried oregano
- ½ teaspoon paprika
- ½ teaspoon chili flakes
- ½ teaspoon garlic powder
- 4 eggs

Directions:

Healthy Liver For Life And Cookbook

- Toss butter in the pan and melt it.
- Then add chopped mushrooms and bell pepper.
- Roast the vegetables for 5 minutes over the medium heat.
- After this, add red onion and stir well.
- Sprinkle the ingredients with garlic powder, chili flakes, dried oregano, and dried thyme. Mix up well
- After this, add tomato paste and water.
- Mix up the mixture until it is homogenous.
- Then add fresh parsley and dill.
- Cook the mixture for 5 minutes over the medium-high heat with the closed lid.
- After this, stir the mixture with the help of the spatula well.
- Crack the eggs over the mixture and close the lid.
- Cook shakshuka for 10 minutes over the low heat.

Nutrition:

calories 123, fat 7.5, fiber 1.7, carbs 7.8, protein 7.

Ham Spinach Ballet

Servings: 4

Cooking Time: 40 Minute

Ingredients:

- 4 teaspoons cream
- ¾ pound fresh baby spinach
- 7-ounce ham, sliced
- Salt and black pepper, to taste
- 1 tablespoon unsalted butter, melted
- Preheat the oven to 360 degrees F. and grease 2 ramekins with butter.
- Put butter and spinach in a skillet and cook for about 3 minutes.
- Add cooked spinach in the ramekins and top with ham slices, cream, salt and black pepper.
- Bake for about 25 minutes and dish out to serve hot.
- For meal preparation ping, you can refrigerate this ham spinach ballet for about 3 days wrapped in a foil.

Nutrition:

Calories: 188 Fat: 12.5g Carbohydrates: 4.9g Protein: 14.6g Sugar: 0.3g Sodium: 1098mg

Ultimate Liver Detox Soup

Servings:5

Cooking Time:20 Minutes

Ingredients:

- 2 tablespoons extra-virgin olive oil
- 1 cup chopped shallot
- 1 tablespoon grated ginger
- 2 cloves garlic, minced
- 4 cups homemade chicken broth
- 1 medium golden beet, diced
- 1 large carrot, sliced
- 1 cup shredded red cabbage
- 1 cup sliced mushrooms
- a handful of pea pods, halved
- 1 hot chili pepper, sliced
- 1 cup chopped cauliflower
- 1 cup chopped broccoli
- 1 bell pepper, diced
- A pinch of cayenne pepper
- A pinch of sea salt
- 1 cup baby spinach
- 1 cup chopped kale
- 1 cup grape tomatoes, halved

Directions:

- In a large skillet, heat olive oil until hot but not smoky; sauté in shallots, ginger and garlic for about 2 minutes or until tender; stir in broth and bring the mixture to a gentle simmer.
- Add in beets and carrots and simmer for about 5 minutes. Stir in hot pepper, cauliflower and broccoli and cook for about 3 minutes. stir in bell pepper, red cabbage, mushrooms, and peas and cook for 1 minute.
- Remove from heat and stir in salt and pepper. Stir in leafy greens and tomatoes and cover the pot for about 5 minutes. Serve.

Nutrition:

3g carbs 10g fat 12g protein 165 Calories

Breakfast Beans (ful Mudammas)

Servings:1

Cooking Time:10 Minutes

Ingredients:

- 1 (15-oz.) can chickpeas, rinsed and drained
- 1 (15-oz.) can fava beans, rinsed and drained
- 1 cup water
- 1 TB. minced garlic
- 1 tsp. salt
- 1/2 cup fresh lemon juice
- 1/2 tsp. cayenne
- 1/2 cup fresh parsley, chopped
- 1 large tomato, diced
- 3 medium radishes, sliced
- 1/4 cup extra-virgin olive oil

Directions:

1. In a 2-quart pot over medium-low heat, combine chickpeas, fava beans, and water. Simmer for 10 minutes.
2. Pour bean mixture into a large bowl, and add garlic, salt, and lemon juice. Stir and smash half of beans with the back of a wooden spoon.
3. Sprinkle cayenne over beans, and evenly distribute parsley, tomatoes, and radishes over top. Drizzle with extra-virgin olive oil, and serve warm or at room temperature

Nutrition:

35g carbs 30g fat 20g protein 460 Calories

Chicken Stir Fry With Red Onions & Cabbage

Servings: 3

Cooking Time: 10 Minutes

Ingredients:

- 550g chicken, thinly sliced strips
- 1 tablespoon apple cider wine
- 2 teaspoons balsamic vinegar
- Pinch of sea salt
- pinch of pepper
- 4 tablespoons extra-virgin olive oil
- 1 large yellow onion, thinly chopped
- 1/2 red bell pepper, sliced
- 1/2 green bell pepper, sliced
- 1 tablespoon toasted sesame seeds
- 1 teaspoon crushed red pepper flakes
- 4 cups cabbage
- 1 ½ avocados, diced

Directions:

1. Place meat in a bowl; stir in rice wine and vinegar, sea salt and pepper. Toss to coat well.
2. Heat a tablespoon of olive oil in a pan set over medium high heat; add meat and cook for about 2 minutes or until meat is browned; stir for another 2 minutes and then remove from heat.
3. Heat the remaining oil to the pan and sauté onions for about 2 minutes or until caramelized; stir in pepper and cook for 2 minutes more.
4. Stir in cabbage and cook for 2 minutes; return meat to pan and stir in sesame seeds and red pepper flakes. Serve hot topped with diced avocado

Nutrition:

283.6 Calories 11.5g fat 31g carbs 10.9g protein

Chocolate Muffins

Servings:7

Cooking Time:30 Minutes

Ingredients:

- 2 eggs
- 1 tablespoon olive oil
- 1 cup milk
- 2 cups whole wheat flour
- 1 tsp baking soda
- ¼ tsp baking soda
- 1 tsp cinnamon
- 1 cup chocolate chip

Directions:

- In a bowl combine all dry ingredients
- In another bowl combine all dry ingredients
- Combine wet and dry ingredients together
- Fold in chocolate chips and mix well
- Pour mixture into 8-12 preparation ared muffin cups, fill 2/3 of the cups
- Bake for 18-20 minutes at 375 F, when ready remove and serve

Nutrition:

2g carbs 6g fat 10g protein 100 Calories

Deviled Eggs

Servings: 8

Cooking Time: 20 Minutes

Ingredients:

- 8 eggs
- ½ cup Greek Yogurt
- 1 tablespoon mustard
- 1 tsp smoked paprika
- 1 tablespoon green onions

Directions:

- In a saucepan add the eggs and bring to a boil
- Cover and boil for 10-15 minutes
- When ready slice the eggs in half and remove the yolks
- In a bowl combine remaining ingredients and mix well
- Spoon 1 tablespoon of the mixture into each egg
- Garnish with green onions and serve

Nutrition:

35g carbs 30g fat 20g protein 460 Calories

Brown Rice And Grilled Chicken Salad

Servings: 3

Cooking Time: 10 Minutes

Ingredients:

- 300g grilled chicken breasts
- 3/4 cup brown rice
- 1 1/4 cup coconut water
- 1 teaspoon minced garlic
- 2 tablespoons teriyaki sauce
- 1 tablespoon extra-virgin olive oil
- 2 tablespoons cider vinegar
- 1 small red onion, chopped
- 5 radishes, sliced
- 1 cup broccoli, chopped
- Dash of pepper

Directions:

- Cook rice in coconut water following package instructions. Remove from heat and let cool completely, and then fluff with a fork.
- Whisk together garlic, teriyaki sauce, extra virgin olive oil, and vinegar. Stir in red onion, radishes, broccoli and rice. Season with pepper and stir until well blended. Serve with grilled chicken breasts.

Nutrition:

283.6 Calories 11.5g fat 31g carbs 10.9g protein

Banana Quinoa

Servings:4

Cooking Time:12 Minutes

Ingredients:

- 1 cup quinoa
- 2 cup milk
- 1 teaspoon vanilla extract
- 1 teaspoon honey
- 2 bananas, sliced
- ¼ teaspoon ground cinnamon

Directions:

- Pour milk in the saucepan and add quinoa.
- Close the lid and cook it over the medium heat for 12 minutes or until quinoa will absorb all liquid.
- Then chill the quinoa for 10-15 minutes and place in the serving mason jars.
- Add honey, vanilla extract, and ground cinnamon.
- Stir well.
- Top quinoa with banana and stir it before serving.

Nutrition:

Calories 279, fat 5.3, fiber 4.6, carbs 48.4, protein 10.7

Toasted Crostini

Servings: 4

Cooking Time: 15 Minutes

Ingredients:

- 12 slices (1/3-inch thick) whole-wheat baguette, toasted
- Coarse salt and freshly ground pepper
- For the spread:
- 1 can chickpeas (15 1/2 ounces), drained, rinsed
- 1/4 cup olive oil, extra-virgin
- 1 tablespoon lemon juice, freshly squeezed
- 1 small clove garlic, minced
- 2 tablespoons olive oil, extra-virgin, divided
- 2 tablespoons celery, finely diced, plus celery leaves for garnish
- 8 large green olives, pitted, cut into 1/8-inch slivers

Directions:

- In a food processor, combine the spread ingredients and season with salt and pepper; set aside.
- In a small mixing bowl, combine 1 tablespoon of olive oil and the remaining ingredients. Season with salt and pepper. Set aside.
- Divide the spread between the toasted baguette slices, top with the relish. Drizzle the remaining1 tablespoon of olive oil over each and season with pepper. If desired, garnish with the celery leaves. Serve immediately.

Nutrition:

603 Cal, 3.7 g total fat (3.7 g sat. fat), 0 mg chol., 781 mg sodium, 483 mg pot, 79.2 g carb.,9.6 g fiber,6.8 g sugar, 19.1 g protein.

Quick Cream Of Wheat

Servings:1

Cooking Time:12 Minutes

Ingredients:

- 4 cups whole milk
- 1/2 cup farina
- 1/2 tsp. salt
- 3 TB. sugar
- 3 TB. butter
- 3 TB. pine nuts

Directions:

1. In a large saucepan over medium heat, bring whole milk to a simmer, and cook for about 4 minutes. Do not allow milk to scorch.
2. Whisk in farina, salt, and sugar, and bring to a slight boil. Cook for 2 minutes, reduce heat to low, and cook for 3 more minutes. Stay close to the pan to ensure it doesn't boil over.
3. Pour mixture into 4 bowls, and let cool for 5 minutes.
4. Meanwhile, in a small pan over low heat, cook butter and pine nuts for about 3 minutes or until pine nuts are lightly toasted.
5. Evenly spoon butter and pine nuts over each bowl, and serve war

Nutrition:

3g carbs 10g fat 12g protein 165 Calories

Pan-fried Chicken With Oregano-orange Chimichurri & Arugula Salad

Servings: 3

Cooking Time: 5 Minutes

Ingredients:

- 1 tablespoon orange juice
- 1 teaspoon orange zest
- 1 teaspoon dried oregano
- 1 small garlic clove, grated
- 2 teaspoon apple cider vinegar
- 1/2 cup chopped parsley
- 1 1/2 pound chicken, cut into 4 pieces
- 1 tablespoon lemon juice
- A pinch of pepper
- 1/4 cup olive oil
- 4 cups arugula
- 2 bulbs fennel, shaved
- 2 tablespoons whole-grain mustard

Directions:

1. Make chimichurri: In a medium bowl, combine orange zest, oregano and garlic. Mix in vinegar, orange juice and parsley and then slowly whisk in ¼ cup of olive oil until emulsified. Season with black pepper.
2. Sprinkle the chicken with lemon juice and pepper; heat the remaining olive oil in a large skillet and cook the chicken over medium high heat for about 6 minutes per side or until browned.
3. Remove from heat and let rest for at least 10 minutes. Toss chicken, greens, and fennel with mustard in a medium bowl; season with salt and pepper.
4. Serve steak with chimichurri and salad. Enjoy!

Nutrition:

3g carbs 10g fat 12g protein 165 Calories

Pineapple, Macha & Beet Chia Pudding

Servings:4

Cooking Time:10 Minutes

Ingredients:

- 1 cup chia seeds
- 1 teaspoon raw honey
- 2 cups almond milk
- 1 teaspoon matcha green tea powder
- 2 tablespoons fresh beetroot juice
- 1 whole pineapple
- 1 cup freshly squeezed lemon juice
- 1 knob of fresh ginger
- Toasted almonds and figs to serve

Directions:

1. Green Chia pudding layer:
2. Add another half each of chia seeds, raw honey, almond milk, and matcha green tea powder to the blender and until very smooth; transfer to a bowl.
3. Beetroot layer: blend together beetroot and ginger with the remaining chia seeds, raw honey, vanilla, and coconut milk until very smooth; transfer to a separate bowl. In a food processor, puree the fresh pineapple until fine.
4. To assemble, layer the chia pudding in the bottom of serving glasses, followed by the pureed pineapple and then the beetroot layer. Top with figs and toasted almonds for a crunchy finish.

Farro Salad

Servings:2

Cooking Time:4 Minutes

Ingredients:

- 1 tablespoon olive oil
- A pinch of salt and black pepper
- 1 bunch baby spinach, chopped
- 1 avocado, pitted, peeled and chopped
- 1 garlic clove, minced
- 2 cups farro, already cooked
- ½ cup cherry tomatoes, cubed

Directions:

Heat up a pan with the oil over medium heat, add the spinach, and the rest of the ingredients, toss, cook for 4 minutes, divide into bowls and serve.

Nutrition:

calories 157, fat 13.7, fiber 5.5, carbs 8.6, protein 3.6

Apple Oatmeal

Servings: 3

Cooking Time: 8 Minutes

Ingredients:

- 1/2 tsp ground cinnamon
- 4 tbsp. fat free vanilla yogurt
- 1 1/2 cups quick oats
- 1/4 cup maple syrup
- 3 cups apple juice
- 1/4 cup raisins
- 1/2 cup chopped apple
- 1/4 cup chopped walnuts

Directions:

- Combine your cinnamon and apple juice in a saucepan and allow to boil.
- Stir in your raisins, maple syrup, apples and oats.
- Switch the heat to low and cook while stirring until most of juice is absorbed. Fold in walnuts, serve and top with yogurt.

Nutrition:

242 Calories 25g carbs 12g fat 13g protein

Citrus Chicken With Delicious Cold Soup

Servings:3

Cooking Time:30 Minutes

Ingredients:

- 2 tablespoons extra-virgin olive oil
- 500g ounces chicken breast
- 1 teaspoon fresh rosemary
- 1 lemon, sliced
- 1 orange, sliced
- For the Cold Soup:
- 2 tablespoons apple cider vinegar
- 1/4 cup green pepper, chopped
- 1/4 cup cucumber, chopped
- 1/2 cup onion, chopped
- 3 cloves garlic, minced
- 1 cup stewed tomatoes

Directions:

1. Generously coat chicken with extra virgin olive oil and cover with rosemary, lemon and orange slices. Bake in the oven at 350°F for about 30 minutes.
2. In a blender, blend together all the soup ingredients until very smooth and then serve with chicken and cooked brown rice.

Nutrition:

3g carbs 10g fat 12g protein 165 Calories

Vegetable Omelet

Servings:3

Cooking Time:10 Minutes

Ingredients:

- Egg whites – 4
- Egg – 1
- Chopped fresh parsley – 2 Tablespoons.
- Water – 2 Tablespoons.
- Olive oil spray
- Chopped and boiled red bell pepper – ½ cup
- Chopped scallion – ¼ cup, both green and white parts
- Ground black pepper

Directions:

1. Whisk together the egg, egg whites, parsley, and water until well blended. Set aside.
2. Spray a skillet with olive oil spray and place over medium heat.
3. Sauté the peppers and scallion for 3 minutes or until softened.
4. Over the vegetables, you can now pour the egg and cook, swirling the skillet, for 2 minutes or until the edges start to set. Cook until set.
5. Season with black pepper and serve.

Nutrition:

Calories: 77 ,Fat: 3g ,Carb: 2g ,Phosphorus: 67mg ,Potassium: 194mg ,Sodium: 229mg ,Protein: 12g

Crunchy Peach, Cranberry And Flax Meal Super Bowl

Servings:3

Cooking Time:10 Minutes

Ingredients:

- 10 ounces frozen cranberries
- 10 ounces frozen peaches (or mangoes)
- 1 cup almond milk
- 1 cup water
- 1/4 cup flax meal
- 1/3 cup chia seeds
- 1/4 cup raw honey
- Toasted walnuts and toasted coconut for serving

Directions:

- In a blender, combine water and peaches and blend until very smooth; transfer to a bowl.
- Blend almond milk and cranberries until very smooth.
- In a serving bowl, mix together the fruit purees and then stir in flax meal, chia seeds, and raw honey until well combined.
- Let sit for at least 10 minutes before serving. Serve topped with toasted walnuts and toasted coconut

Nutrition:

242 Calories 7g Carbs 19g Fat 12g Protein

Olive Frittata

Servings:5

Cooking Time:15 Minutes

Ingredients:

- 9 large eggs, lightly beaten
- 8 kalamata olives, pitted, chopped
- 1/4 cup olive oil
- 1/3 cup parmesan cheese, freshly grated
- 1/3 cup fresh basil, thinly sliced
- 1/2 teaspoon salt
- 1/2 teaspoon pepper
- 1/2 cup onion, chopped
- 1 sweet red pepper, diced
- 1 medium zucchini, cut to 1/2-inch cubes
- 1 package (4 ounce) feta cheese, crumbled

Directions:

- In a 10-inch oven-proof skillet, heat the olive oil until hot. Add the olives, zucchini, red pepper, and the onions, constantly stirring, until the vegetables are tender.
- Ina bowl, mix the eggs, feta cheese, basil, salt, and pepper; pour in the skillet with vegetables. Adjust heat to medium-low, cover, and cook for about 10-12 minutes, or until the egg mixture is almost set.
- Remove from the heat and sprinkle with the parmesan cheese. Transfer to the broiler.
- With oven door partially open, broil 5 1/2 from the source of heat for about 2-3 minutes or until the top is golden. Cut into wedges.

Nutrition:

288.5 Cal, 22.8 g total fat (7.8 g sat. fat), 301 mg chol., 656 mg sodium, 5.6 g carb.,1.2 g fiber,3.3g sugar, 15.2 g protein.

Pancakes

Servings:4

Cooking Time:30 Minute

Ingredients:

- 1 cup whole wheat flour
- ¼ tsp baking soda
- ¼ tsp baking powder
- 2 eggs
- 1 cup milk

Directions:

- In a bowl combine all ingredients together and mix well
- In a skillet heat olive oil
- Pour ¼ of the batter and cook each pancake for 1-2 minutes per side
- When ready remove from heat and serve

Nutrition:

2g carbs 6g fat 10g protein 100 Calories

Heavenly Egg Bake With Blackberry

Servings:4

Cooking Time:15 Minutes

Ingredients:

- Chopped rosemary
- 1 tsp lime zest
- ½ tsp salt
- ¼ tsp vanilla extract, unsweetened
- 1 tsp grated ginger
- 3 tbsp coconut flour
- 1 tbsp unsalted butter
- 5 organic eggs
- 1 tbsp olive oil
- ½ cup fresh blackberries
- Black pepper to taste

Directions:

- Switch on the oven, then set its temperature to 350°F and let it preheat.
- Meanwhile, place all the ingredients in a blender, reserving the berries and pulse for 2 to 3 minutes until well blended and smooth.
- Take four silicon muffin cups, grease them with oil, evenly distribute the blended batter in the cups, top with black pepper and bake for 15 minutes until cooked through and the top has golden brown.
- When done, let blueberry egg bake cool in the muffin cups for 5 minutes, then take them out, cool them on a wire rack and then serve.
- For meal preparation ping, wrap each egg bake with aluminum foil and freeze for up to 3 days.
- When ready to eat, reheat blueberry egg bake in the microwave and then serve.

Nutrition:

Calories 144, Total Fat 10g, Total Carbs 2g, Protein 8.5g

Walnuts Yogurt Mix

Servings: 6

Cooking Time: 10 Minutes

Ingredients:

- 2 and ½ cups Greek yogurt
- 1 and ½ cups walnuts, chopped
- 1 teaspoon vanilla extract
- ¾ cup honey
- 2 teaspoons cinnamon powder

Directions:

In a bowl, combine the yogurt with the walnuts and the rest of the ingredients, toss, divide into smaller bowls and keep in the fridge for 10 minutes before serving for breakfast.

Nutrition:

calories 388, fat 24.6, fiber 2.9, carbs 39.1, protein 10.2

Asparagus With Egg

Servings: 4

Cooking Time: 20 Minutes

Ingredients:

- 1 lb. asparagus
- 4-5 pieces prosciutto
- ¼ tsp salt
- 2 eggs

Directions:

- Trim the asparagus and season with salt
- Wrap each asparagus pieces with prosciutto
- Place the wrapped asparagus in a baking dish
- Bake at 375 F for 22-25 minutes
- When ready remove from the oven and serve

Nutrition:

35g carbs 30g fat 20g protein 460 Calories

Pear Oatmeal

Servings: 4

Cooking Time: 20 Minutes

Ingredients:

- 1 cup oatmeal
- 1/3 cup milk
- 1 pear, chopped
- 1 teaspoon vanilla extract
- 1 tablespoon Splenda
- 1 teaspoon butter
- ½ teaspoon ground cinnamon
- 1 egg, beaten

Directions:

- In the big bowl mix up together oatmeal, milk, egg, vanilla extract, Splenda, and ground cinnamon.
- Melt butter and add it in the oatmeal mixture.
- Then add chopped pear and stir it well.
- Transfer the oatmeal mixture in the casserole mold and flatten gently. Cover it with the foil and secure edges.
- Bake the oatmeal for 25 minutes at 350F.

Nutrition:

calories 151, fat 3.9, fiber 3.3, carbs 23.6, protein 4.9

Conclusion

Eating can improve and alleviate symptoms of liver cirrhosis. It is important to stay hydrated with water, juice or other fluids because dehydration will cause a build up of toxins in the body. A diet low in fat but high in protein and carbohydrates help maintain proper weight while giving essential nutrients for fighting off infection. The list goes on! But one thing that you need to know about your liver is that it's still working hard even if you have lost 80% function due to alcohol abuse.

Cirrhosis is an irreversible, chronic liver disease that can lead to complete organ failure. The cirrhosis diet plays a major role in the course of this condition and there are both eating tips for people with liver cirrhosis as well as information on how the functions of the liver work. You're not alone; many people suffer from this disease without knowing they are living with it until later stages when the risks increase considerably, so let's take care of our livers so we can live better!

www.ingramcontent.com/pod-product-compliance
Lightning Source LLC
Chambersburg PA
CBHW070920080526
44589CB00013B/1374